I0491463

TOP 5 MOST POWERFUL
LAW OF ATTRACTION MANTRAS

*A 21-day practice for spiritual and
physical healing, success, money, and
getting literally everything you want*

DR. JENNIFER VIVIAN

TEXT COPYRIGHT © [DR. JENNIFER VIVIAN]
ISBN: 9798675892099

TABLE OF CONTENT

Book Description

I am very lucky as I have known mantras and used them to change everything in my life, and I would like to share this wonderful thing with all of you.

Are you struggling with illness and/or discomfort? Are you dealing with health issues such as insomnia, sleeping disorder, anxiety, depression, infertility, or any other mental physical disease?

Do you want your family members to be safe and secured from the aforementioned and any other illness? Do you want you and your family to live a life of total happiness, fulfillment, joy, sound health, and success?

You're reading the very book that will show you how.

If there's one thing you're required to know is that we live in a world that is made up of sound and vibration at its well-refined level. Everything from trees, fields, and even people produce distinct sound and vibrations. The high qualities that you reveal in life have their vibrations.

Have you heard about the mantra? Well, this refers to a certain sound or vibration that comes with known results. When you begin to chant out loud or even silently, you can bring transformation, healing, and also awakening in your life and to those around you.

In this book, you're going to find out;

- What mantra is.
- How you can chant a mantra.
- The power behind mantras and the general benefits of mantras.
- Why and also just how mantras assist us to heal.

- The practice principles of mantras.
- The five sacred mantras that will certainly bring you healing and happiness.
- Step by step how to practice mantras – a very simple way to really help in some particular situations:
  - ➢ Mantra to heal insomnia, sleeping order, depression, anxiety, stress
  - ➢ Mantra to heal infertility
  - ➢ Mantra to get a safe pregnancy and delivery
  - ➢ Mantra to protect your kids and your family from dangers
  - ➢ Mantra for urgent help in dangerous situation
  - ➢ Mantra to find a suitable job
  - ➢ Mantra to find a good partner
  - ➢ Mantra to restore a happy marriage
  - ➢ Mantra in daily practice to get wealth, health, success and long life.

Once you have grasped the wisdom of Universe through Law of Attraction Mantra, it is bound to turn your life around for the better. That's what this book is all about: healing, curing, improvement, destiny transformation, and a sense of internal peace.

So, what are you still waiting for? Journey with me as I take you on this healing trip.

Happy reading!

Introduction

It is quite unfortunate that despite having the arrival of modern medication as well as healing approaches to medical recoveries, there is still a higher contour in the variety of emerging illnesses. What is sad is that the price of medical care which is increasingly difficult to obtain for the common man. Every minute, there's a spike in the price of drugs or health care insurance.

Are you suffering from a condition that modern medicine has no cure for? Well, you might be in luck!

The Universe is one of the best (if not the best) as well as a cost-free physician that will certainly bring you back to full recovery. Believe me, unlike other modern doctors, you will certainly not spend a penny if you picked the Universe as your physician, regardless of just how ill or just how much discomfort you are undergoing.

By mantra practice, we become a physician for ourselves and also for our families, even when we are healthy or when we go under severe conditions and discomforts.

We are different people dealing with unique difficulties every day. These difficulties pose a threat to our mental stability, leaving us with worries and concerns. We are always caught up in a battle of life, trying to satisfy our aim for existence. Noble development, success, and satisfaction of worldly satisfaction that will not only bring us freedom and earn us spiritual fulfillment. It is the actual reason that we come to tap into the Universe's power.

Being a mom of two, I have discovered to value the relevance of mantras in operating the Universe's power in my personal life, marital relationship, and also parenthood. Life can be tough on the home front if you're a parent or being responsible for others. Things like sickness, clinical depression, household breakdowns, childbirth, being a wife/husband, as well as monetary responsibilities can take a toll on you and make you feel out of your element. If you are not mindful, you may wind up with depression.

The concept and relevance of mantras may be strange to Westerners. Yet, it has been practiced by numerous Eastern people for thousands of years. These deeply-spiritual exercises called mantras are extremely straightforward to practice. They can also give you the desired result and even more.

What's more? You can practice mantras whenever you carrying out your normal daily chores such as food preparation, working, caring for your children, or doing homework. So, don't worry if you are very busy. Some mantras don't take you any more time. Why not incorporate it with western medications in healing?

Personally, if there's one thing that assisted me in my healing process, it is mantras. You may be thinking, "But what are mantras anyway?" Mantra is simply a set of syllables and also short words that you chant repetitively; whether loudly or quietly. It is among the most simple techniques for Law of Attraction that someone can apply to their daily lives. It has unmeasurable power. It is something that will not only aid you to locate your true self but will aid you to envision as well as develop the future you've always fantasized about.

Millions of people before us have successfully mastered

and utilized mantras to sustain their health and wellness routines, and improve their lives as a result. Some have efficiently utilized it to transform their minds and take advantage of the endless power of their psyche, paired with the intervention of their magnificent exterior surroundings. What you need to keep in mind is that while exercising mantra, a crucial component is sincerity and complete faith! Mantra has been credited to cancer cells remissions, enhanced life expectancy, riches, healing as well as healing from defilements.

You need to understand is that mantras have the Power of Healing, whether physical or psychological. On the other hand, if you are in good condition, it will certainly assist shield you from different threats and also impending illness. It is what will certainly offer you a long life, joy, and even lasting wealth.

It also can secure you as well as your family members from all conditions, all-natural disasters, dangers, and also deaths. What is more is that you can practice mantras whenever you are doing such things as cooking, working, or taking care of your kids. As well as if you can invest 30 minutes daily to practice mantras incorporated with the meditation technique, it will aid you the best within a very short time.

Mantras likewise can assist you to take care of the material worries and needs of life. We all have a pressing desire to make changes in our lives. A few of us want new friends. Others desire a new job or occupation. Some desire to be abundant. Some want to be successful in their work and even the home front. Many of us have dealt with health issues or know a person who has. People deal with economic issues and many life changes. We have needs that can be as basic as a brand-new car or a brand-new home or as made complex as smoothing out some twisted family members mess. Many of us also want aid in handling our emotions as well as internal lives. We come across situations that produce knee-jerk reactions that we would love to avoid. We become annoyed, depressed, mad, and envious. Many of us want our children to be safe as well as devoid of all difficulties in life. Some would love to have a happy marriage.

These issues can throw us into depression, anxiousness, stress, and anxiety that medicines cannot help. Mantra practice can help you get quality regarding your life, your objective, and yourself.

There are times where we'd be in positions to help others. The problem then becomes how we would do so. A relative or coworker might be in some trouble, or we want to be able to contribute to the good of our neighborhood or the globe-- if only we understood what to do. Mantra can aid you to locate the best course of action for efficient modification. The relatively straightforward tool of mantra can aid you with all the problems and also the difficulties you require to encounter. Even though mantra is ancient in the beginning, you can use it to practically any type of contemporary concern with good results. Whatever it is that you are going through today, know that it is nothing that mantras cannot help you accomplish.

There are different types of mantra and countless publications for directing mantra practice. This book will give you a clear cut overview to practice 5 chosen mantras to enhance all types of issues in your life. This publication is likewise valuable to understand just how to use those mantras practice to cure certain conditions.

Inside this book, I will guide you in detail just how to practice mantras properly for healing, controlling depression-anxiety-stress, treating sickness, defense, bring in money as well as success in many areas, and also getting anything you want. You likewise discover just how to use them to heal some particular diseases on your own and your household, and also conquer some life problems.

Some mantras can be chanted aloud or in silence while you are doing your work: as you wash dishes, as you meditate, as you cook, as you look after your kids, and as you go to bed. Healing Mantras currently make this sound medication readily available to everyone:

- Mantra for healing the inability to conceive as well as for a successful developing a wellness a child

- Mantras for Maternity, Birth, Protection your children and household as well as Beyond

- Mantra for urgent help

- Mantra for being employed

- Mantra for effective business

- Mantra for a great partner, excellent companion, happy marital relationship

- Mantra for mentally and also literally for yourself and others

- Mantra for overcoming depression, anxiousness, and also tension, consisting of Bipolar disorder, Post-traumatic anxiety disorder, Boundary personality disorder, Postpartum clinical depression.

- Mantra for healing sleeplessness and sleeping disorders

- Mantra for the daily practice for defense, healing and also a healthy and delighted life

And also the most wonderful thing is that, if you do specifically what I direct in this book, you can see the wonders after 21 days. Open yourself to the possibility and also the power of mantras. Embrace these five powerful mantras.

Settle down, grab a glass of water, and enjoy this wonderful and soul-lifting read.

Chapter 1: What Is Mantra?

A mantra describes a set of expressions that are repeated with well-known effects. It can either be a single word or a long-phrase.

Words like "mantra" in itself are stemmed from Sanskrit, which means an idea that underlies an activity of speech. Integrating mantra and meditation can assist to find as well as discover our Universe's power which can alter your life.

What we will be concentrating on in this book are some of the most powerful mantras that are still practiced today.

You may be thinking, "however why we utilize mantras?" Well, to recognize mantras, it is essential that you think about it as a form of meditation. To put it simply, they are made use of as a method of motivating a proper placement between the inner and exterior globes.

When incorporating this practice, you can choose to speak out loud, read, sing, or chant mantras. When you chant out loud and even silently, you can bring change, healing, and awakening in your life.

Practicing mantra is the same as a meditation integrated with the power of sound to aid you to heal all your issues. In other words, mantras are time-focused and lasting.

Trust me, it's a lovely feeling to tap into the power of the Universe as well as utilize it to drive your life.

Chapter 2: How Do You Chant a Mantra?

Initially, you may feel that utilizing mantra at the beginning is self-exploratory. However, with time you will realize that it involves a lot of practice. Nonetheless, to start chanting mantras, the first thing you ought to do is to pick whether you would love to practice it formally or informally.

Formal practice

Formal mantra practice refers to a form of meditation. It is one that you exercise each time when nobody will disrupt you. As a result, you can dedicate 10-15 mins every day to do your Mantra.

Begin by determining which is the most comfortable place is that you can do your mantra. After that settle on your own by either sitting down quietly. Then spend a minute to absorb a deep breath, close your eyes, and also begin concentrating on what is essential to you. Start to pray for your demands as you chant your mantra.

One thing that you need to note is that you do not need to do this loudly for it to have an impact. When you do it silently, the study shows that this has a much more effective impact in itself.

For that reason, create a special me-time to freely explore the deeper meaning of the mantras. Begin by thinking of each expression or word you recite and after that, please give yourself time to ruminate and moil over each word to tap into their Power.

If you do not have sufficient time to commit to formal practice, then you can exercise your Mantra informally while working or doing your everyday jobs.

Informal practice

Unlike the formal practice where you spend private time to doing your Mantra, informal practice is suitable for when you do not have that time to do so. This implies that, once you have actually prayed, you can start chanting your Mantra at any time. You could be doing your Mantra while preparing food, cleaning, driving, or doing any other thing.

This kind of mantra practice offers an excellent opportunity for the modern individual with an ever active schedule. This is the kind of Mantra that is frequently instructed across the world. When you are around people would not like to disrupt them, all you need to do is whisper your sounds sub-vocally. Believe me; you will be surprised how much different personal mantra will carry your very own life.

You'd find that it is useful when you find yourself in a scenario that calls for an individual mantra. All you've got to do is repeat your Mantra as often as you can under your breath. You can additionally pair it with brief mindfulness and self-alertness to ensure that your experience is grounded. In case you are caught up in an urgent scenario that needs the aid of Mantra, concentrate on what matters to you the most, and you will be surprised at just how the mere practice works like magic.

If you're thinking that mantra through mumbling isn't a thing, it is. Trust me that it isn't just mumbling!

Chapter 3: The Power and Basic Benefits of Mantras

There are a lot of advantages that mantra practice has on your daily life. As human beings, we are prone to a lot of problems. Nevertheless, with the preparation work of mantras, mindfulness, and also meditation, you obtain protection from all the concerns that life contends you. This is because mantras have the power to set your mind free, recover, protect your brain, as well as enable it to remain mindful throughout the day.

According to research, proofs of this originated from centuries and unscientific documents that demonstrate the advantages of mantras. For example, research performed by the China Agricultural College revealed that the practice of mantras has an effect on crops and also increased the outcome by over 15%.

What is even intriguing is the reality that individuals that practice lots of farming and also horticulture utilize relaxing music in their mantras.

Lee Mirabai, a critically acclaimed writer, and artist, disclosed that she makes use of mantras with her garden to counteract the result of air pollution. She additionally utilizes it to nullify the impacts of heavy metals on the plants and also the environments. What is much more intriguing is the fact that plants have been revealed to thrive with certain sound vibrations.

Well, health modifications are undoubtedly reasonable. Yet with the practice of mantra meditation, you can dramatically reduce your stress levels. This will, in turn, improve your healing from various health conditions. When this is paired with faith, there is a sensible degree of recovery that belief produces.

Chanting the mantra as part of your daily routine can prevent you from distress and harmful occurrences. At the very least, the mantra can considerably aid you to conquer all the storms in your life. This allows the light to come shinning again.

For many years, I have actually discovered many mantras for addressing life's troubles. To give you some suggestions on how this can work, I wish to inform you just how a mantra assisted me with a specifically difficult time.

When giving birth to my children 5 years ago, I had actually fulfilled severe postpartum anxiety from dealing with my kids as well as financial concern without any work. I desired to have a full-time task with revenue of regarding US$1,000 each month. I obtained lots of tasks however no reaction from them.

My marriage was really difficult as a result of the arguments with my spouse regarding financial stress, and also problems regarding motherhood. I came under stress and anxiety. The good news is, I have discovered mantras before. I established a goal of finding a steady task to relieve clinical depression and also receive a living wage. During that time, I was a bit skeptical as well as thought that with my qualification, I cannot do anything to gain US$ 1,000 each month.

But I disregarded those uncertainties, just chanting mantra and asked the Universe for my need. I also went surfing on the web to discover tasks. I figured out a way to practice mantra seriously at any moment. I needed a substantial amount of time for my mantra practice.

Given that several analytic mantras are basic in nature, the mantra I chose was one for the elimination of obstacles: Great Compassion mantra. This mantra (which will certainly be discussed in chapter 6) is universally acknowledged as very reliable for removing obstacles of all kinds.

Before the practice of this mantra daily, I ask for stable, lasting, and appropriate work. I defined the task thoroughly that it would appropriate for my ability, the location of the job was near my home as well as the salary is US$1,000.

I continued to apply for other jobs and also repeated the mantra as much as I could daily, in some cases quietly, often aloud. I needed to spend practically of day to care for my children, so I repeated this mantra while executing family duties, strolling, consuming, or preparing food. When going about my day, I would maintain the mantra going as long as I could. If I was with other individuals, I would certainly chant silently. If I was alone, I would chant softly aloud. Despite just how hectic, I attempt to chant Great Compassion mantra at the very least half an hour per day. At the end of the day, I prayed for all people all over the world and made a request to the Universe for a peaceful world.

After 3 weeks, this wonderful thing occurred to me. I obtained an invitation from a friend's project without having to send my application. They sent me a deal of US$ 1,000 each month for editor placement. It was the very first time I saw the magic of mantra. As well as even more unbelievably, the task that I passed was practically exactly what I explained before.

Utilizing mantra to get gainfully employed typically takes 3 weeks - an extremely short time. For various other problems, mantra practice might take a longer time to get the outcome, depends on your full trust in mantra's power and also your practice.

Chapter 4: Why Mantra Can Assist Us Heal And Recover?

Like earlier discussed, the study of mantras originated from the classic Eastern design of just how the Universe works. According to this design, the Universe carries energy, which functions as the most essential thing when it concerns manifesting the type of life we want. This is done by taking advantage of the power of sound resonances.

You may be pressed with this question: "What does sound have to do with anything?" Well, one thing that you need to remember is that sound is regularity as well as a resonance that has a significant impact on water. On the other hand, human beings are largely made up of water. This describes the reason mantras have a favorable effect on human life along with that of plants.

It might appear foolish to you initially to accept the fact that sound can change one's life. Well, among the questions that I have listened to many people asked is just how in the world mantra can set off protection, recovery, and good luck, whether there is faith or not.

Something that you need to keep in mind is that when you do away with unfavorable energies in your life, you make room for positive ones to enter your scenario. This is the reason the Mantra functions! However, one of the most vital inquiries once more is, "How does mantra work?"

There are several ways in which mantra functions. On one end, it makes use of sound resonances, something that has been proven over centuries of spiritual experiments. It likewise works by utilizing the all-natural psychological problem of the mind.

For many years, there has actually been proof that points at mantra generating a transformed state of mind, which goes a long way in bringing recovery with anxiety decrease.

Fortunately, when you practice mantra, you have a chance to attain liberty from fate. This is mostly based upon the belief that the reason we remain in our current conditions; whether in health and wellness or individual life, is because of negative fate that results from our previous actions.

Mantra removes the negative karmic causes of illness and cultivates the causes for well-being. Simply put, mantra works off unfavorable karma by way of mindfulness and sacred sounds that link us with the divine globe.

The reality shows that in the period of practice mantra, we always alter our mind and also alter our action right into much better actions. This aids us to change our therapy to others. It also assists to unlock the power in our inner mind.

The other point to note is that when you chant mantras, it has a significant influence on all forms of fate. Therefore, this helps in conquering what you may have inadvertently created with a lack of knowledge in your past life. However, you have to recognize that mantras do not need to translate into actual meanings. To put it simply, the spiritual syllables OM, HUM, and AH do not always mean anything; therefore, they are taken into consideration sacred with high degrees of significance.

Chapter 5: Mantra Practice Principles

Set your goal target and ask for your desire daily as detailed as possible

One of the vital things when exercising mantra is having an objective in mind. It doesn't matter if you are doing it for the sake of happiness, success, dedication, healing, or mindfulness. Before you can begin chanting, you need to spend some time to establish an objective, and then you can go ahead and start chanting.

Be clear and concise about what you want. For every duration of practice, simply try to focus on one wish. You may have different aspirations, but surely one of them is more important. Focus on that.

If you do not recognize exactly what you want, you can really take steps to do it. To share something, you must understand what you want.

That suggests you need to recognize the specifics quite possibly, describing the attributes as if your expression was specifically developed for you.

The mantra's principal works as the Law of Attraction. Please note that the primary catches that people fall under when they ask the Universe for something are that they are not 100% sure what they desire as well as why. You must ask for something from the Universe that is being accurate and also clear regarding what you desire. To avoid deep space taking a long time to think about what you want, you should describe your wishes in as much detail as possible.

For instance.

If you intend to amass wealth, what does wealth mean to

you? How much of it do you want?

If you desire a job, please describe the work information: kind of task, wanted salary, office space, number of days of rests annually, etc.

If you wish to take care of every problem, please explain your problem is in as much detail as possible and how you desire it to vanish.

If you intend to resolve the issue of any individual, please define her/his problem. Do not fail to remember to provide her/his information such as full name, date of birth, home, etc.

If you intend to buy a new home, please describe exactly the worth of the house you want, its location, its structure and also design, etc.

If you need love, what kind of partner do you want? Please note that you define thoroughly what you desire, you do not have to spend a lot of time to get it since the Universe does not require to take a long time to presume.

Find a quiet area where you will not be distracted by outdoors or within the noise. Close your eyes and concentrate entirely on simply the one great thing you want.

Daily, you send out demands to the Universe—in addition to your subconscious mind—in the form of thoughts: what you consider, check out, talk about, as well as offer your attention to.

Ask the Universe what you desire once a day every day; you have to make your demands clear and concise.

Repetition of mantra as much as you can (a

minimum of 108 times each day)

If you need to create a condition for healing, curing, mindfulness, meditation, and getting what you desire, you need to focus on what it is that you wish to attain from the mantra. The very best method to accomplish this is through repeated mantra. It is essential that you recite the mantra at a minimum of twenty-one recitations. However, in a meditation session, what is recommended is a minimum of 108 mantras.

But why 108? Well, 108 repetitions are symbolic for the 108 things that afflict life. There are at least six different forms of illusions, namely; mind, body, eyes, tongue, nose, and ears. Each of these things happens in three ways; present, past and the future.

Additionally, these times take place by two conditions of the heart; a pure and an impure spirit. They also possess three sentiments namely indifference, like, and dislike. When you multiply all these together, you get 108, a number that defines the number of mantra repetitions to be performed and has been held significant by so many religious traditions. That said, what you will notice is that so many mantra practitioners will meditate on several thousands of mantras a day.

Daily practice

This is the best approach when it comes to mantra practice. The main reason why you need to practice mantra each day is to maintain a consistency that convinces the mind that you are putting first your divinity.

When you prioritize God at the top of your to-do list, what

you are merely doing is allowing him to change the world through you. This is precisely how you can bring peace into the world. When you devote at least a few minutes to an hour each day, to do mantra, you are merely giving God 10% of your time, and He will also give Himself to you.

Place of practice

One thing that you need to understand about the mantra is that it is a sound vibration that transcends the place you choose for practice. If you are too busy, you also focus on chanting mantra when you do your work. However, for the best effective result from the mantra's power, you should find a quiet place while practicing mantra. It will help you focus on your wish and each sound of mantra to get its power.

Just sitting down alone somewhere, away from the noise, and focusing your attention on either your breath or a mantra of some sort. It is similar to a method of meditation. Please keep it simple so that you can do it at any time.

Chant with sincerity and full faith: Just ask and let everything go by itself

You MUST practice it with absolute trust in the mantra's power.

Put your trust in the mantra the same way you put your trust in the Universe. Trust that the Universe has the best Power. Trust it completely 100% (even not 99%) that the Universe will bring you the best results.

A crucial step that is often overlooked by people is trusting the Universe to do right by you, even if it doesn't seem that way on the surface. Just think that you are putting your wish in the best power.

How to realize that you don't trust 100% in mantra's power? That is when you work toward your goal, you may give out the question if mantra actually works. You might lose your belief in mantra practice. You count day by day to see if your wish becomes true but it seems that it doesn't. When you question the mantra's power, you're invariably saying that the mantra doesn't work.

The limiting beliefs in mantra's power have kept many people from success, wealth and happiness. If it is the same to you, firstly you have to change your mindset and put the absolute belief in mantra's power while practicing it.

JUST ASK AND LET IT GO. What if I tell you that you will get the miracle after 21 days of chanting mantra? Will you practice mantra and count day by day to wait for the result? After 20 days, you begin to doubt that mantra doesn't work as everything wouldn't go well. If you do that, it means that you don't put your full trust in mantra.

Don't wait and don't count day by day. You need to believe that once you have sent your wish into the Universe, it will get back to you in perfect time. Please remember that you are seeking a response from the other side. So just relax and rid your mind of worries.

When practicing mantra, you have to ensure that you are doing it with sincerity and not just as a chore that you must do. You have to ensure that you remain mindful of the mantra, its sounds, and the techniques that you employ during meditation. Your full commitment should be on the practice and not as a ritual. That way, you can effect change in your life and your destiny.

To Mala or not to Mala

Mala refers to straightforward aids of counting at a basic degree. If you need to concentrate on your practice of rule, you can include mala to compute.

Nevertheless, one thing that you have to keep in mind is that as soon as you start using mala, you need to treat them with the utmost regard. In this manner, you can highly reinforce the mantra practice, though it is not required.

Be Thankful

When you are offered the things you requested, be appreciative of them and also show your gratefulness in your activities.

And also, do not forget to give thanks for whatever else you have, whether you asked for it or otherwise.

Do not fail to remember to pray for others, not for only you.

Based on the above principles, right here's a simple structure of workouts you can use to begin.

1. Locate a quiet place, close your eyes, and also focus on slowing down your breathing.

2. Make your demand

3. Repeat a mantra.

4. Dedication

It's also a means of meditation. The routine practice of mantra will aid clear your mind of diversions, clean your thoughts, and also boost your spiritual link. It restores the spirit, relaxes the body, as well as soothes the spirit. It also helps to raise the efficiency of rule practice.

Chapter 6: Five Sacred Mantras And How To Practice Each Of Them Step By Step

The practice of mantra today is done with so much devotion as it was many centuries ago. Here are the five most potent mantras in the world that I have selected for you to practice.

1. Medicine Buddha Mantra

I put this mantra as the first because it's the mantra for all things in our lives: health, longevity, curing mental and physical diseases, riches, success, happy marriage, happiness. This is one of the most popular mantras believed to bring about the healing energy for pain, illness, stress, anxiety, and other diseases.

Medicine Buddha is the best doctor and his mantra is said to be the best treatment remedy in the entire Universe. It is open for use by anyone that wishes to bring the healing energy of the medicine.

Medicine Buddha mantra is one of the most sacred mantras in healing. We can practice the Medicine Buddha mantra for healing ourselves or healing someone we care about who is ill. In Medicine Buddha sutra, Medicine Buddha promises to help remove pain, suffering, disease, and disabilities of all living beings, as well as boost good health and wealth. So, by Medicine Buddha mantra practice, we can cure ourselves of all diseases and get all our needs in our life.

Millions of people have practiced Medicine Buddha mantra for thousands of years. Medicine Buddha practice will not replace modern medical treatment but complement it.

In the West, modern medical focuses on the treatment of physical symptoms, while traditional Eastern meditation focuses more on the solutions for the mental roots of illness. It is our luck if we can access both of the two methods and combine them properly for our health.

This mantra will not only eliminate suffering and problems you might have but also benefits animals at all times, even when they are healthy and whole. It also brings about success in all areas of your life, allowing for growth, enlightenment, and happiness. If you are in pain, you can alleviate it by reciting this mantra.

How to practice Medicine Buddha Mantra that combined with meditation:

Getting Started

Find a quiet place to recite the mantra. The place may be anywhere provided that it is away from noise and distractions.

MAKING YOUR REQUEST

Ask Medicine Buddha to remove pain, cure disease, or anything you need at that time: money, success, happy marriage, the best partner, or long life. Please, describe your desire in detail so that your praying will be more effective.

RECITING MEDICINE BUDDHA'S MANTRA

Here is Medicine Buddha's mantra which is in Sanskrit:
"Tayata, Om Bekanze Bekanze,
Maha BeKanze BeKanze
Radza Samudgate
Soha."

This is pronounced (we will pronounce as below when

reciting this mantra):

"Tie-ya-tar, om beck-and-zay beck-and-zay,
ma-ha beck-and-zay beck-and-zay
run-zuh sum-oon-gut-eh
so-ha."

DEDICATION

End your session with a dedication. The most important thing is that you should dedicate the merit of mantra to all beings, not to yourself only.

You can make your dedication such as, "By this practice of Medicine Buddha, I ask for the world to be peaceful, for all living beings to be free from pain, illness, and suffering, for sound health to be restored, and for all men to see the light."

When you do this, you will draw the power from these words *"Tayata Om Bekanze Bekanze Maha Bekanze Radza Samudgate Soha"* and receive your great healing.

OTHER NOTICE

To practice it daily, you have to be ready to do it formally. In other words, you have to devote time out of your busy schedule to practice this mantra. Once you have identified a quiet place where you can pray, chant this mantra at least 108 times a day. Once you are done, pray for others as well to benefit from it.

But we cannot count the times when chanting as our minds have to focus on the mantra. So, try using a counting machine or practice in 30 minutes.

However, if you are too busy to do this formally, you can also do it informally. Try to do it at least 108 times per day by calling the name of Medicine Buddha *"Namo Medicine*

Buddha." You can call His name "*Namo Medicine Buddha*" in silent or speaking it out. And then, at the end of the day, you conclude your praying with a dedication as above - it is very important.

2. Great Compassion Mantra

Although Medicine Buddha mantra has the power to give us all that we need, there are also some mantras to practice more in certain circumstances.

The Great Compassion mantra is the second most chanted mantra that millions of people around the world chant. They sing Maha Karuna Dharani, the highest Compassion mantra of Avalokitesvara. This form of the mantra is famous for its purification, healing, and protection benefits.

This mantra has 84 lines, and you can easily incorporate into your routine.

This mantra has a wide range of benefits that each one of us will appreciate. Some of the immediate benefits you will draw according to sutra teachings, and commentaries include healing, protection, and purification from negative karmas.

These 15 kinds of unfortunate deaths are from; starvation or poverty, imprisonment, hostile enemies, military battles, fierce animals (such as tigers and wolves among others), the venom of poisonous animals (like snakes, scorpions, and black serpents), drowning or burning, poison, mediumistic insects, evil diseases that bind the body, nightmares by evil people, madness/insanity, suicide, natural disasters (like falling trees or landslides), or deviant spirits and evil ghosts.

Instead, they will enjoy such good tidings as; meeting

good friends, being born in good countries, being born at good times, having a good king, living with a kind and harmonious family, having a pure and full heart, will find what they desire. Their wealth will not be plundered, the dragons, good spirits and gods will always watch over them. They will find awakening to the true meaning of Dharma. They will see Buddha and hear of Dharma in their places of birth. They will not violate prohibitive precepts. Their body organs will always be complete. They will have the help and respect of those around them, and will always have an abundance of wealth.

In addition to general benefits, this mantra also has the power to help us in some circumstances (finding a job, find the way to have a baby naturally). We will discuss this in the next chapter.

So, how do you practice this mantra daily?

For this particular mantra, all you need to do is chant about 5-7 times. However, one thing that is important to note here is that the most effective way is to chant is 21 times each day, coupled with meditation and formal practice.

Steps:

GETTING STARTED

Find a quiet place to recite the mantra. The place may be anywhere provided that it is away from noises or distractions.

MAKING YOUR REQUEST

Ask for what you need as detailed as possible.

RECITING MANTRA

Here is the mantra which is in Sanskrit:

1. *Namah Ratna Trayaya.*
2. *Namo Ariya.*
3. *VaLokitesvaraya.*
4. *Bodhisattvaya.*
5. *Mahasattvaya.*
6. *Mahakaruniakaya.*
7. *Om.*
8. *Sarva Rabhaye.*
9. *Sudhanadasya.*
10. *Namo Skrtva i Mom Ariya.*
11. *Valokitesvara Ramdhava.*
12. *Namo Narakindi.*
13. *Herimaha Vadhasame.*
14. *Sarva Atha. Dusubhum.*
15. *Ajeyam.*
16. *Sarva Sadha. Nama vasatva.*
17. *Namo Vaga.*
18. *Mavadudhu. Tadyatha.*
19. *Om. Avaloki.*
20. *Lokate.*
21. *Karate.*
22. *Ehre.*
23. *Maha Bodhisattva.*
24. *Sarva Sarva.*
25. *Mala Mala*
26. *Mahe Mahredhayam.*
27. *Kuru Kuru Karmam.*
28. *Dhuru Dhuru Vajayate.*
29. *Maha Vajayate.*
30. *Dhara Dhara.*
31. *Dhirini.*
32. *Svaraya.*
33. *Cala Cala.*

34.Mamavamara.

35.Muktele.

36.Ehi Ehi.

37.Cinda Cinda.

38.Arsam Pracali.

39.Vasa Vasam

40.Prasaya.

41.Huru Huru Mara.

42.Huru Huru Hri.

43.Sara Sara.

44.Siri Siri.

45.Suru Suru.

46.Bodhiya Bodhiya.

47.Bodhaya Bodhaya.

48.Maitriya.

49.Narakindi.

50.Dharsinina.

51.Payamana.

52.Svaha.

53.Siddhaya.

54.Svaha.

55.Maha Siddhaya.

56.Svaha.

57.Siddhayoge

58.Svaraya.

59.Svaha.

60.Narakindi

61.Svaha.

62.Maranara.

63.Svaha.

64.Sirasam Amukhaya.

65.Svaha.

66.Sarva Maha Asiddhaya.

67.Sarva

68.Cakra Asiddhaya
69.Svaha.
70.Padmakastaya.
71.Svaha.
72.Narakindi Vagaraya.
73.Svaha
74.Mavari Samkraya.
75.Svaha.
76.Namah Ratnatrayaya.
77.Namo Ariya
78.Valokites
79.Varaya
80.Svaha
81.Om. Siddhyantu
82.Mantra
83.Padaya.
84.Svaha.

DEDICATION

End your session with a commitment and pray for all, such as, "By practice Great Compassion mantra, I ask for the world to be peaceful, for all living beings to be free from pain, illness, and suffering, for health to be restored and perfect enlightenment."

OTHER NOTICE

To exercise it daily, you have to prepare to do it formally. Simply put, you need to commit time out of your active timetable to exercise this mantra. When you have recognized a silent location where you pray, chant this mantra at the very least 7 times a day. The very best is 21 times a day. As soon as you are done, wish others too to benefit from it.

No need to translate or comprehend the definition of

mantras as it has the sacred meaning.

3. Mantra to secure kids and also maternity

If you are an expectant mother, this mantra is the very best choice for you to practice every single day. The advantage with this mantra is that it provides protection to kids against any type of harm, and also gives them a lengthy as well as delightful life. These mantras lines are;

"Padmi padmi-devī

Kṣīni kṣīni kṣemin,

Jūre jūra jūrī
Hūrā hūrā,
Yu rī, yu ra, yu rī,
Para pari-muñca,
Chide bhide
Bhañje
Māthe
Chida-kare
Svāhā"

Steps:

- Begin by looking for an area that allows you to concentrate on your mantra.

- Close your eyes, take a deep breath to unwind and start paying attention to each word that you chant.

- Ask for what you want. This mantra specifically for safeguard your kids and to make certain they are constantly healthy and balanced, happy and safe.

- After that start chanting this mantra for at least 108 times.

- End your session with dedication and praying for all, such as, "By practicing this mantra, may I ask for the world to be peaceful, and all live beings specifically children worldwide be without pain, condition, and suffering, as well as always be safe."

4. Lotus Sutra Mantra

It is likewise described as a heart sutra mantra or prajnaparamita mantra. The verse of this mantra is *"Gate gate paragate parasamgate. Bodhi! Svaha!"*

Something with this mantra is that it supplies superb illumination that sheds light on one's life to damage the darkness that had taken over before. Consequently, by stating this mantra, you are ruining the darkness, ignorance, and also afflictions in your life in unlimited previous karmas.

Steps:

- Start by finding a location that is suitable for you to focus on your mantra.

- Then close your eyes, absorb a deep breath to loosen up and also start focusing on each word that you chant.

- After that start praying for somebody or something else as well as keep chanting this mantra for a minimum of 108 beads.

- End your session with a devotion and praying for all, such as, "By practicing this mantra, may I ask for the world to be peaceful, for all live beings be free from pain, illness, and suffering, and quickly restore health and perfect enlightenment."

5. Namo Guan Shi Yin Pu Sa Mantra

This is one more mantra that is associated with Guan Yin.

You can exercise this mantra informally daily whenever you are doing your work. It is critical that you do at least 108 times for this mantra.

Steps:

- Locate a suitable area for you to concentrate on your mantra.

- After that, close your eyes, absorb a deep breath to relax as well as begin taking notice of each word that you chant.

- Start by chanting three times of *"Namo Guan Shi Yin Pu Sa."*

- Then, ask for your wish. After that, keep chanting *"Namo Guan Shi Yin Pu Sa"* for a minimum of 108 times.

- End your session with dedication and pray for all, such as, "By practicing *"Namo Guan Shi Yin Pu Sa"* mantra, I ask for the world to be peaceful, for all live beings be free from pain, illness, and suffering, sound health and perfect enlightenment."

Some of the benefits of this mantra are the reality that it permits you to receive magnificent security from all-natural catastrophes, risks (diseases), and also tragedies.

Furthermore, it uses filtration of impediments that arise from greed, temper, as well as deceptions. It additionally provides one with guts as well as compassion they require to get over barriers in their lives.

I put this mantra right here because it is different from other mantras. It is very valuable to aid you in emergency conditions if you practice it daily such as earthquakes, plane crashes, emergency crashes, or fire accidents.

We will go over more regarding this in the next chapter.

Chapter 7: How Do You Apply Mantra Practice To Treat Some Particular Diseases and Obtain A Far Better Life?

One question I listen to many individuals asking is how they can apply different types of mantra to heal their ailments so that they can bring joy right into their lives. Well, the answer is chanting the mantra will assist you to attain that, and also the outcomes are evident within 3 weeks to 3 years.

All mantras support you in healing and also locate what you want in life. Yet using a proper mantra in a certain situation will make it advertise all its efficiency. Right here are just how to select a proper mantra in some specific situations to obtain its support quickly.

Mantra for Healing Infertility as well as an effective giving birth to a Healthy Child

I will give you something unique that you can do together with taking medicines-- a mantra to help you receive expectantly.

Pregnancy is a divine stage in a female's life, and also if she is voluntarily taking the step to be a mother, she is overjoyed when she finds out about the tiny infant in her womb.

While some womens conceived and give birth to their kids easily, there are others who are yet to bear a kid.

Practicing mantra can help you get conceive successfully even if you are infertile. The inability to conceive is specified as trying to be pregnant (with frequent sexual intercourse) for a minimum of a year without any success. Whether male or female infertility, or a combination of the two impacts millions of couples in the United States. An estimated 10 to 18 percent of couples have trouble getting pregnant or having successful childbirth.

The inability to conceive results from female elements regarding one-third of the time as well as male factors about one-third of the time. The reason is either unidentified or a combination of man and female factors in the remaining situations.

The inability of women to conceive can be difficult to diagnose. There are lots of readily available treatments, which will certainly depend upon the root cause of infertility. Therapy may make you become anxious and filled with stress. The mantra always functions well with you even if you still have not obtained an excellent rise from modern medical therapy for a long time.

If you're hoping to be pregnant, don't leave it to the luck. You can use a mantra to turn your scenario around. No matter if your test report says, there is a mantra that you can chant to hold your baby in your arms, quickly.

Which mantra should you make use of in this circumstance?

The solution is for you to chant Great Compassion mantra with outright belief for a minimum of 21 times daily. Exercise all steps (which discussed in the previous Phase) with full belief until you obtain the bright side. The results are seen in 3 weeks to 3 years. This period is generally for all mantras in healing. However, to my experience, the wonder will certainly occur after 3-6 months.

The most important in this period is that you need to relax. Just doing Great Compassion practice (21 times per day in a quiet place and end your practice each day by dedication) and let it go. The result will come to you in the best time.

Mantra for Safe Maternity, Birth, Security your children and Beyond

Chanting mantra while pregnant helps to procure a favorable impact on the growth and development of babies in the womb. Mantra is shown to be really effective for expectant women even in this materialistic world. It creates a high resonance, a spiritual sound, as well as deep, caring tranquility for yourself as well as your growing infant. Chanting mantras can boost your heart and you may feel a close link to particular mantras during pregnancy.

A mantra is a powerful device for tranquility and happiness during significant changes in maternity. As a mother, you should chant them throughout your pregnancy for healthy mom and healthy baby, as well as for very easy delivery.

For your pregnancy protection, pray for simple delivery as well as to guarantee your kids' health and wellness. Chant the adhering to below mantra:

"Padmi padmi-devī
Kṣīni kṣīni kṣemin,
Jūre jūra jūrī,
Hūrā hūrā,
Yu rī, yu ra, yu rī,
Para pari-muñca,
Chide bhide

Bhañje
Māthe
Chida-kare
Svāhā"

Complying with mantra has solid healing powers that will certainly sustain you as well as protect your infant from the womb to the future. This mantra likewise assists to prevent losing the unborn baby.

Chanting this mantra every day for at the very least 108 times.

Mantra brings about positive thinking that has the power to help your infant's development and growth. Mantra silence the mind and open the heart, producing unified problems for both mother and child. Even from inside the womb, your infant can hear you and would love the sound of your voice.

Chanting mantras will offer your infant the happiness of hearing his/her mommy's voice. An excellent mantra can do wonders, so keep chanting them daily during your maternity. It is the best means to invite a brand-new spirit to this globe!

You can additionally use this mantra when your baby is birthed to protect her/him in the future.

Mantra for Help in urgent situations

I will show you a pointer to make use of mantra in really immediate minutes which are when we were in a collapsed aircraft or a sunk ship, or a fire or flooding.

In those moments, we need to keep one's cool. Do not panic, temporarily put the life and death aside, simply focus on chanting "*Namo Guan Shi Yin Pu Sa*" constantly with complete belief. It makes sure that the threat will turn good, all individuals will relieve from the yoke.

Momentarily of urgency, attempt to recite "*Namo Guan Shi Yin Pu Sa*" as high as possible. There will certainly be hope. Simply chanting with a single-minded idea, regarding it with full faith, the threat will certainly turn safety.

In Eastern culture, *Guan Shi Yin Pu Sa* can help us in urgent situations. Imagine that if we were in a bus and the driver lost his control of the bus, and the bus was going down to a deep abyss. In that very dangerous moment, call Guan Shi Yin Pu Sa's name, surely all people would be risk-free.

During the critical hour of emergency, reciting "*Namo Guan Shi Yin Pu Sa*" one time equals a hundred thousand times in the normal time. So, you will see the miracle.

If you can chant this mantra daily, it would be great as it could help you to away from danger and disaster.

Every day you can chant "*Namo Guan Shi Yin Pu Sa*" at any time when doing anything. This mantra is the first mantra that I learn in my life. When I was a little child, my mom taught me to chant "*Namo Guan Shi Yin Pu Sa*" at any time in the day. My mom had full faith in Guan Shi Yin Pu Sa and also practice the mantra every day.

In 1990, a huge flood came to my hometown. Before the night of the flood, my sister and I were sleeping. In the middle night, my mom called my dad and us to wake up. My mom said that she dreamed that a flood was coming soon. We had to move away immediately. We also informed our neighbors to go away. All of us were safe before the flood came.

My mother always recites "*Namo Guan Shi Yin Pu Sa*" at any time, so when we encounter incurable diseases and disasters, we always are safe.

Mantra for Being Employment

If you are searching for work, you should begin by hoping and after that chanting Great Compassion mantra at the very least 21 times every day.

The most effective method is to take a minimum of 30 minutes daily to practice it officially by requesting your dreaming work, meditation, and chanting that mantra. Adhere to precisely all steps that I discussed to this mantra in the previous chapter.

Mantra for Successful Business and Wealth

For a successful business, you need to exercise formally with asking, meditation as well as chanting Medicine Buddha 108 times each day after praying for it. Do the same when you need wellness, lengthy life, and also outstanding levels of prosperity.

Mantra for a Perfect Lover, Great Partner, Happy Marriage

If you need joy in your marriage or to rekindle your lovemaking, wish a wanting companion or marital relationship and after that repeat Medicine Buddha mantra 108 times daily.

If you have a poor relationship in your marriage, practice Medicine buddha's mantra daily will aid you to realize your error. You always see that the errors belong to you. It would make you transform your treatment.

If you wish to produce an abundance of love in your life, after that concentrate on love. Be the love you intend to attract.

Come to be extra caring and charitable with others as well as with yourself. By creating the vibration of love, you will instantly draw more love right into your life.

Focus on whatever it is that you intend to create more of in your life, and bear in mind to be happy for that which you currently have.

Gratitude itself is a type of abundance, as well as the vibrational regularity of gratefulness and appreciation will immediately attract much more to be grateful for.

Mantra for Healing as well as Curing for others

The best way is to ask them to practice Medicine Buddha practice with meditation for at least 108 times per day. If they are in serious disease and they cannot practice the mantra by themselves, you can do it for them. Prepare a glass of water and put it beside you.

You should use your left hand to make a shape with your fingers pointing towards the glass of water. You chant 108 times Medicine Buddha and then, let the patient drink that glass of water. This time, water is considered as medicine by Medicine Buddha.

Please do it daily and don't forget to ask for healing and curing their disease before practicing mantra.

Mantra for who are in Depression, Anxiety and Stress that drugs cannot help them

Mantras can help anyone who is in clinical depression, anxiousness and also stress and anxiety, Bipolar affective disorder, Post-traumatic anxiety condition, Multiple personality disorder, Postpartum clinical depression. The most effective way is to ask practice Medicine Buddha practice with meditation for at the very least 108 times daily. Medicine Buddha is very handy in these instances.

Mantra for Recovery Insomnia and also Sleeping Disorder

The very best way is to practice Medicine Buddha mantra with meditation for at least 108 times per day. Medicine Buddha is the best mantra to recover psychological diseases, so it is the best medicine for sleeping problems.

Don't fail to remember to follow all steps when practicing this mantra, including concluding your session with a dedication for all beings in the world.

Mantra for daily practice for Protection, Healing and a Healthy and Happy Life

Even if you are healthy and balanced, please maintain to chant Medicine Buddha's mantra daily as a meditation to keep your life constantly be in the manner in which you want.

It's fantastic if you can invest half an hour daily to chanting Medicine Buddha's mantra. Simply a little time every day to get a wonderful life that you want. Why not?

Conclusion

There are countless stories of individuals using mantra to attain success, wonders, and many other things that they never ever thought was possible. I understand that everyone has various concerns they are dealing with and desires they wish to attain.

Whatever the case, it is important to bear in mind is that mantras are for everybody. No matter the physical or spiritual issues, practice mantra combined with meditation. It doesn't matter whether you practice Islam, Christianity, Buddhism, any other religious beliefs or you are just a normal person. The Law of Attraction states that you will draw in right into your life whatever you concentrate on. Mantra also works in the same way with The Law of Attraction, so mantra constantly benefits you.

Understand that chanting mantra is one of the vital spiritual disciplines that will certainly enhance your paying attention skills, mindfulness, increased power, and help you remain sensitive to other people. It is with chanting mantra that you obtain the possibility to express dedication, tranquility, gratitude, and compassion. This is just how you introduce light into your life to destroy the darkness within you.

Whatever you do, bear in mind to put your full faith in your recitations of mantra. If you pair your practice of mantra with your full belief in it, you will certainly have a solid will to go after your life's objectives.

When you have a sound body as well as a calm mind, your chanting of mantras will certainly be worthwhile. And when you're totally free from any concern, you will begin to realize that light has entered your life together with joy, pleasure, and gratification.

So, what are you still waiting for? Beginning chanting mantra today and sharing mantras with others, you'd understand the many benefits of it in no time.

Best of luck!